CALMNESS SERIES

Slimming Down and Loving It!

3 Steps to Reboot Your Mind and Reshape Your Body

by Inessa Zaleski, DD, CMCH, RM

COPYRIGHT PAGE

Dedication

This book was made possible because of continuous support from my immediate family. Their unwavering faith in me kept me going through many revisions and rewrites.

I dedicate this book to them and to my first teachers. Thank you for your knowledge, wisdom, support and love.

Contents

INTRODUCTION

I remember countless hours sitting at the kitchen table observing my grandmother in her domain. She was an amazing craftswoman - creating delicious healthy dishes with only the few limited ingredients that were available to us in Russia. The first decade of my life was spent with her, as my mother worked two jobs. I am forever grateful to her - my first teacher - who started my education about the importance of proper nutrition and healthy eating habits.

I am fortunate to have had a wonderful second teacher: my mother. Armed with vast medical knowledge, she educated me about the direct correlation between proper nutrition and health. She went out of her way to ensure I ate only healthy, nutritional, homemade dishes that she created with dedication, thoughtfulness and - most importantly - love. After working most weeknights until 7pm, she stayed up late making meals for the family and got up early to buy fresh hot rolls for us to take to school.

My father was another great first teacher, I learned a lot from him about causation, and emotional connections to food. I was fascinated to learn that experiences in early childhood can profoundly influence eating habits and food choices. I'm forever grateful to him for raising my awareness.

Since then, and throughout my adult life, I'm continuously amazed and fascinated observing the direct (and sometimes immediate) connection between what we ingest and our overall well-being. This curiosity led me on the path to discovery that ultimately created this effortless, step-by-step guide for healthy eating that you're holding today.

Foreword

The fact that you are reading this book is your first step toward conquering not only the challenge of losing weight, but you will soon realize that you can also overcome other emotional challenges that cause people to be 'stuck'. Dr. Inessa illuminates a path that shows us how to 'un-stick' ourselves from habits and mind-sets that keep us from being the best we can be.

You are about to embark on an Incredible Journey of Self-Mastery that is easier than you ever imagined.

Dr. Inessa's wonderful system lays it out, step-by-gentle-step, and all you have to do is DO IT!

The first "baby step" is to know that you can!

Congratulations! Your new life has just begun!

Rita Graham
Singer, Actor, Author
Former Ray Charles Raelette, Star of the magical, musical film, "We Are Kings" 2013, Author of the suspense novel, Karma Rising
(Amazon.com, Kindle, Nook, AuthorHouse Publishing)

Unhealthy eating habits that had survived decades of good intentions and firm resolutions began to change. Daily I find myself rejuvenated and energized as Inessa helps me to rediscover my birthright of wholeness and well-being!
--- Michael, USA

I definitely have changed my eating habits. I sit down, enjoy what I eat, eat smaller portions, and I do not take seconds. Most important in my case: I have given myself permission to read without eating at the same time. Finally, I am walking at least 30-45 minutes a day…
--- Betty, USA

I had great reservations…. but was willing to try anything to help me lose weight. Losing 17 pounds in 5 weeks without "being on a diet" made me a believer. I feel energetic without feeling any deprivation. I don't know why it works, just that it does! The relaxation technique was an added bonus…….
--- Linda, USA

Dear Dr. Inessa, thank you for helping me do the impossible: have the best body ever! Now I have a much stronger and younger looking body then I had 30 years ago, when I was 18 years old! Your method works magic!
--- Nicole, France

GETTING STARTED

The call came late on a Friday afternoon.

"I am looking for Dr. Inessa Zaleski…." the voice sounded faint and uncertain, "My doctor told me to call you…"

I didn't immediately respond, as I was still trying to decipher the caller's gender.
The voice hesitated a moment longer before continuing, "My doctor said you can help people like me . . . "
And after a deep breath: "I need to lose 300 pounds."

Local physicians had been referring their patients to me for years for things like weight control, stress management and smoking cessation; however, this was different. Recently, I've experienced an influx of obese patients.

Obesity is defined as having a high body to fat index. As it turns out, obesity isn't just an issue around here – it's global. Worldwide, the fifth-leading risk factor for death is obesity. [1]

Astoundingly, according to the World Health Organization (WHO), health issues rooted in obesity kill 2.8 million people every year. While world hunger used to present the greater threat, now the 1.6 billion people who are obese (with a Body Mass Index above 30%) or overweight (a BMI of 25-29.9%) outnumber the malnourished and starving almost 2-to-1.

In 2008, one third of American adults were obese, and close to 70% were overweight. Just two years later, the WHO stated that 64% of American adult females were overweight, as well as 74% of American adult males. [2]

Being overweight or obese is quickly becoming more of a concern. In fact, every year in America we spend more than $150 billion on health-care aimed at this very issue! [3]

The United States isn't the only place affected by obesity. Pacific Island countries like Samoa and Tonga have much higher obesity levels than the US. In the Middle East, Saudi Arabia and the United Arab Emirates have a higher obese population than the U.S. too, and Iraq is close behind. Even the percentage of Mexican men and women considered obese recently overtook the U.S. Worldwide over 500 million adults are categorized as *obese*. And that's not the worst of it.

A staggering 43 million pre-school children are obese or overweight. [4] Obesity is the second highest cause of preventable deaths. [5] *Obesity and its related risks will soon overtake tobacco-use as the number one cause of death.* [6]

Listed below are some diseases and conditions that are commonly a result of being obese or overweight. These conditions are serious and could even be fatal.

1. **High Blood Pressure**- This is the primary cause of death in Americans older than 25. It can possibly stem from quite a few things. Obesity puts people at a greater risk for high blood pressure. Seventy-five million people suffer from hypertension or high blood pressure, which puts them at a major risk for heart disease. [7]

2. **Diabetes**- More than 90% of those with diabetes worldwide have type 2 diabetes. Being obese or overweight contributes to this. A weight loss of just 5-10% can help decrease the risk of developing diabetes by more than 50%. [8]

3. **Heart Disease**- According to the American Heart Association, obesity is a huge risk factor for developing coronary heart disease: increasing risk by up to 72%! [9] Coronary heart disease can lead to stroke or a heart attack.

4. **High Cholesterol Levels**- One of the top causes of heart attacks, a high cholesterol level can be lowered with a proper diet. [10]

5. **Cancer**- According to a study done by the American Cancer Society, it was found that being overweight can increase your chances of developing cancer by 50%. [11]

6. **Infertility**- Obesity has the ability to cause changes in the hormonal levels of women, and this can cause ovarian failure. It isn't just in women: men who are overweight also have a greater chance of developing low sperm motility and a lower sperm count. Losing just 12 to 14 pounds can lower the risks and increase fertility rates. [12]

7. **Back Pain**- Obesity is a major factor contributing to joint and back pain. [13]

8. **Skin Infections**- Creased areas in the skin can lead to skin infections. [14]

9. **Ulcers**- According to a study done by the National Institute of Health (NIH), obesity can be a factor that contributes to developing gastric ulcers. [15]

10. **Gallstones**- The risk of developing gallstones increases when you are severely overweight (especially for women). [16]

11. **Pulmonary Embolisms**- When people are obese it sometimes causes them to reduce their daily activity. After some time of inactivity, a fatal artery blockage can result. [17]

12. **Polycystic Ovarian Syndrome**- This is a condition where cysts painfully burst, leading to further issues in the ovaries. [18]

13. **Gastro-esophageal Reflux Disease**- This happens when juices and acid regularly come up from your stomach and back into your esophagus. This is common for people who are obese. [19]

14. **Fatty Liver Disease**- A reversible condition which occurs when large pockets of fat accumulate in liver cells. [20]

15. **Hernias**- This Latin word means "a rupture," and occurs when tissue punctures through membrane or a muscle. Most commonly it occurs in the abdomen: the wall becomes weak and a defect (or hole) allows certain tissue to poke through. Being overweight substantially increases your risks of developing one. [21]

16. **Erectile Dysfunction**- This is the failure to gain and maintain an erection. It can be caused by a medical problem that is due to being overweight. [22]

17. **Urinary Incontinence**- Losing the ability to control urination is often related to obesity. [23]

18. **Chronic Renal Failure**- Obese people are at a greater risk for kidney failure. [24]

19. **Lymphedema**- Severely obese people can build up lymph fluid in the fatty tissues just under their skin, which can cause long-term physical, *psychological*, and social problems. [25]

20. **Cellulitis**- This infection spreads through different layers of skin and is caused by obesity-related poor lymphatic flow. [26]

21. **Pickwickian Syndrome** (*Obesity hypoventilation* **syndrome**) - Obesity can place an excessive load on the pulmonary system and cause people to fail to breathe rapidly enough, leading to sleep apnea. [27]

22. **Depression**- Obesity can lead to severe depression and a situation where the person will feel miserable constantly. This can lead to thoughts of suicide. [28]

23. **Osteoarthritis**- This is caused by abnormal wear on the cartilage, which most of the time is a result of obesity. [29]

24. **Gout**- When uric acid accumulates in the blood, nerve endings become subject to irritation which causes intense pain. Carrying extra weight makes this more likely to occur and more severe when it does. [30]

Clearly the dangers are staggering!

Excessive weight gain can literally be life threatening. Not only does it pose major physical threats, the emotional and psychological effects of obesity can drastically reduce your quality of life.

The good news is that releasing excess weight and eating healthily will help you to be happy, stay healthy, live longer, and reduce ALL of the aforementioned risks.

Perhaps you are one of the millions of individuals experiencing obesity; perhaps you are like the individual who phoned me displaying great courage as he admitted that he needs to shed 300 pounds. You may be experiencing some of these health issues already. Perhaps you have tried and tried and tried, longing for success, and failed. Perhaps you feel entirely hopeless.

There is hope, my friend. I understand the intense emotions and feelings associated with being overweight, and I can help you. In this book you will find the answers you have been seeking. You can do this. By picking this book up, you have already taken the first step.

Below you will find tools you can begin to use RIGHT AWAY to take charge of your life.
This is the beginning of a whole new you!!!

Before we roll up our sleeves and begin the real work that stands before us, I want to let you know how incredibly proud I am of your decision to take charge of your weight, to take charge of how you look, to take charge of your self-esteem and ultimately, to take charge of your life.

You now have (in your hands) a powerful tool that was perfected over a quarter of a century and that thousands of people around the world are using to help them take control of their weight. This book guides you to take control of your life, providing tools to start using **right away** to help you permanently improve your eating habits. If you follow the suggestions, you will start feeling and seeing the results within a few short weeks!

I expect that everything in this book will be easy for you to follow. All you need is a desire to succeed, a desire to better yourself, and a willingness to follow through. Follow-through is critically important and can be the most rewarding aspect of this journey. And the good news is that although many of us may feel we lack it, the ability to follow through is an integral part of our human nature.

At a family gathering I was fascinated watching my friend's son Joshua (a one-year-old). Although he fell multiple times, that small baby got up over and over and attempted to walk. He was persistent and kept trying. And he'll keep trying until he can successfully remain upright. As we all know, walking will only be the beginning... As this tot grows he will continue walking, increasing in speed until he is able to run. But it took that initial persistence.

Life and circumstances often try to convince us otherwise, but it's a fact that we all possess this innate ability to push through. I challenge you to get in touch with it, to access it, and use it to better yourself - right now, right this second! I believe in you! You will learn to believe in yourself too!

Below is a note I got recently, and if she's had these results then so can you!

> *Dr. Inessa,*
> *I had mixed feelings when I received an invitation to my 20-year high school reunion. Although I was ecstatic to reconnect with my classmates and show off my successful career as partner at one of the largest law firms in Manhattan, I felt a tight knot in the pit of my stomach when I thought of the 100 pounds that I have gained since high school. Over the years I have tried various diets, but was disillusioned with their temporary success. I was committed to doing it right this time, so I followed the advice of a co-worker who recommended calmness.com. When I started listening to your Weight Control package I*

still had my doubts if this was the best way to lose the extra weight, but after easily getting down to my ideal size and keeping it off for over two years, I am happy to report feeling stronger, happier and much healthier. As a busy professional, I enjoy the fact that I can go to your site and consistently get a high quality product that does the job! Since then I've purchased many of your packages and will be back for more. Thank you!

Susan V., NY, NY

THE FOUNDATION

STEP ONE - A Journey Within: Inner Calmness

I'm sure you are wondering, "How can I truly tackle this challenge? How can I have lasting success?" It's simpler than you may think. Let us begin by going inside.

Inside yourself.

Believe it or not, the first step to taking charge of your weight is to go within yourself. In fact, the first step in tackling any challenge is to get in touch with your calmness. This calmness is sometimes referred to as "your center" or "the zone".

Any great actor or baseball player will tell you that getting in touch with their calmness is what helped them hit that home run or give their best performance.

The more tranquil a man becomes, the greater is his success, his influence, his power for good. Calmness of mind is one of the beautiful jewels of wisdom.
James Allen - British philosopher

Calmness is the cradle of power.
J. G. Holland - American author

Power is so characteristically calm, that calmness in itself has the aspect of strength.
Edward G. Bulwer-Lytton - English novelist

So, why is it beneficial to be calm?
The advantages speak for themselves:

* Increased feelings of well-being
* Better health
* Improved relationships
* Positive outlook on life
* Longevity
* Youthful appearance
* Relaxed disposition
* Stronger heart
* Better sleep and dream recall
* Most likely a normal blood pressure
* Quicker decision making
* Easy elimination
* Clearer vision of the future
* Improved productivity
* Sense of humor
* Much better memory
* Fewer colds and infections

Perhaps Paramahansa Yogananda said it best:
Peace is the altar of God, the condition in which happiness exists.

While the benefits of inner calmness are clearly evident, most people do not achieve this in their lives. The opposite of calm is frazzled and stressed, and a state of inner turmoil. Which one reflects how your life is right now? Are you stressed, rushed, hurried, or simply doing too much?

In a world with people running from activity to activity at a frantic pace, you can still learn to be calm. And although calmness is not an innate quality, it's possible to learn how to get in touch with it and how to embrace it. Every generation strives for calmness and some courageous individuals manage to achieve it. Calmness *is possible!* Thankfully, some of these individuals share their insight with others.

My father used to say to me, "Whenever you get into a jam, whenever you get into a crisis or an emergency, become the calmest person in the room and you'll be able to figure your way out of it".
Rudolph Giuliani *- Former Mayor of New York City*

The more tranquil a man becomes, the greater is his success, his influence, his

power for good. Calmness of mind is one of the beautiful jewels of wisdom.
James Allen - *British philosophical writer*

Any improvement, even a small one, is beneficial. Baby steps are wonderful. That's how we learn to walk, remember? Like watching Joshua... baby steps. So why not improve your calmness the same way? Slowly but surely, you can accomplish this. You can do it. You can gradually integrate calmness into your life. You can have it become part of you, such that when you hear the word *calmness* you instantly find that your muscles are relaxing, stress is instantly abating, your mind is clearing, and you start to feel more and more that you can accomplish anything you put your mind to. I know that you want to feel this way, so let's roll up our sleeves now.

Shall we?

How Do I Achieve Inner Calm?

If you haven't started yet, right now is a wonderful opportunity to incorporate this rewarding and highly beneficial habit into your daily life.

21 DAY CHALLENGE

It's a commonly accepted belief that it takes 21 days to form a habit. This means that if you do something consistently on a daily basis for 21 days you'll find it easier to continue following through after the initial three weeks. That said, I ask that you implement a practice of listening to the Introduction to Deep Calmness script for 21 consecutive days. I am confident that by the end of the 21 days, you will feel better, calmer, and more in control of your life.

With this promise, you are guaranteed to win! While slimming down, consider all that you will gain, including a new lease on life.

I am including the full-length guided visualization script so that you may record it in your own voice. To optimize the experience you may want to practice relaxation before reading the script into your recording device.

In my opinion, relaxation is a necessary part of our daily existence. When you're able to relax yourself, you're able to handle everything that life throws your way. You can start by just taking a few seconds right now.

Please put this book down, relax your arms, close your eyes, and take several deep breaths.

Notice how it feels.
Now doesn't that feel much better?
And as you continue reading this book while you are in a relaxed state, you may notice your mind is much more open to receiving information and remembering the suggestions. These suggestions are easy to follow, and I know you will be able to do it.

I expect that you will find following this book a refreshing and empowering experience. All you need is to make a commitment to invest in yourself, and to carve out some well-deserved time for yourself every day. By investing in your self-development you will find that the benefits accumulate every day!

Finding Time to Relax

When can you find time for yourself?

1. Wake Up Half an Hour Early. - Some people choose to wake up a half hour earlier and use this quiet time for relaxation, centering, and mental preparation for the day.

2. Take a Half Hour After the Kids Go to Bed. - Other people take the time after their kids are in bed to invest in themselves.

3. Eat Lunch in the Park. - Some people grab a sack lunch and go to a park (or its equivalent) to enjoy their "me time" among nature and in peaceful, beautiful surroundings.

4. Take a Walk. - Dr. Raymond Moody (lecturer and best-selling author of books about near-death experiences) shared with me that he cherishes his daily walks so much that when his lecture tour prevents him from enjoying this daily bliss, he compares his withdrawal symptoms to that of an addict.

Find whatever works for you, even if you need to close your bedroom door and put a "Do Not Disturb" sign on it for half an hour! Find your quiet time. Find the time that you can allocate for you and - as much as possible - make it the same time every day.
For the next 21 days, it's important that you find time to relax and use the first script to find calmness.

The purpose and benefits of a script:

This first script is an Introduction to Deep Calmness and its purpose is to train the mind to R E L A X. When you listen to this recording daily for 21 days, you join the tens of thousands of others who have discovered the powerful benefits of daily listening. Additionally, you will be able to train your mind - just like they did, and still do - to relax as deeply as you possibly can.

If, after 10 to 15 days, you want to move on to the next script, you can put this recording aside and start working with the next script. However, for best results listen to this script daily for a minimum of 10 to 15 days. If you are really serious about your desire to take control of your life, I would strongly advise listening to this for the full 21 days. As you remember, many people agree that it takes 21 days to change a habit. This will help you train your mind to be able to relax *at will*. Another benefit of this relaxation is to help you replace stress with tranquility. By learning to calm your mind and body, you will easily minimize internal stress and be able to control how you respond to external stress. This practice will give you a heightened ability to gracefully handle whatever comes your way.

Perhaps your workplace is not the main source of stress in your life. Perhaps your personal life offers a surplus of stressors. Maybe you are doing it all: performing the balancing act of taking care of your children and managing the care of your elderly parents, while developing your career and still looking to spend regular quality time with your spouse. Or maybe your big day is coming. Perhaps you deeply desire to remain calm and feel in control as you walk down the aisle. Maybe you want to approach that cute guy that has been hanging out in your neighborhood or that beautiful woman you met at the hiking club. Maybe you often argue with someone close to you and hope to heal the relationship. It is entirely natural for these types of situations to evoke extreme emotions. Completing the 21 Day Challenge will give you the ability to meet these situations peacefully and confidently.

Go for it. This is the beginning of a completely new, completely calm you. Happy calmness!

DEEP CALMNESS

This chapter contains a relaxation script. Completing the 21 Day Challenge with this script will give you the ability to control how you respond to stressful situations. You will begin to experience greater peace of mind, which will help you gain control over your weight - and ultimately control over your life. You will feel better and start seeing changes in yourself.

Why does it work?

For simplicity of explanation, we are going to compare our mind to a computer. Our subconscious mind performs the instructions that are given to it. It follows the programming that exists in its files.
The following script works like the reboot button on your computer. It will help reset the settings with undesirable files and replace them with the files that you desire.

Ways to use the script:

If you have a recording device handy, you may choose to record the following script in your own voice. Be mindful of your tone, as your ears are sensitive while in the relaxed state and variations in the recording are more obvious when listening. The script below should be recorded using a relaxed, peaceful and calming tone of voice, with pauses at the appropriate times. Keep space for some quiet time within the recording, because the silence is helpful for deepening relaxation. To help you relax even deeper, you may want to mix in peaceful relaxing music.

If you would prefer to move on to the deep relaxation right now, visit *calmness.com/p* to purchase a recording of the script for immediate download. For your convenience, I offer MP3s with voice only or with both voice and background music.

Introduction to Deep Calmness script

Take a deep breath and extend your arms up. Extend your stretch, pushing your arms out even further... feeling your spine stretch... Hold it for as long as it feels comfortable. And as you exhale, slowly lower your arms down... Relaxing your body into complete limpness, like a rag doll... with your legs uncrossed... and your hands at your side or on your lap.

All you need now is to focus on a point of light. It can be any form of light, perhaps a glimmer on a piece of metal or even a bright object. Now... simply look toward the light, toward the source of brightness and allow your eyes to relax...

Allow the muscles around your eyes to relax and allow the muscles in your eyes to relax...
As you look toward the light... toward the source of brightness... just relax your eyes...

Simply allow the muscles around your eyes to relax and allow the muscles in your eyes to relax...

Continue looking toward the light, toward the source of brightness, until your eyes begin to relax ... then allow them to close... Simply allow your eyes to close....... Close your eyes and imagine the light... Imagine the source of brightness... Visualize it in your mind and allow your thoughts to relax...

Allow your body to relax... Relax, relax... and go deeper... Good... Now, I want you to take a deep breath... and let it out completely... relaxing your mind, relaxing your body... and sinking down into this comfortable, relaxed state.

I will be counting from 1 down to number 5 and with each and every number that I say, I would like you to take a deep breath, and each time I say the word "Relax", simply relax and allow the breath to flow out from your body...

One, take a deep breath.... and relax... Two, take a deep breath.... and relax... Three, take a deep, deep breath.... and relax... Four, take a deep breath... and relax, release and relax... Five, take a deep, deep breath.... and relax...
Relax your body, relax your thoughts as you allow this wonderful, comfortable feeling of relaxation flow all the way down to your feet....
Good. Very good.

As you take your next breath, tighten the muscles in your feet, in your calves and in your thighs... hold them... exhale and relax, release and relax... and you can already feel all the large and small muscles of your legs relax. Allow this wonderful feeling of relaxation to flow throughout your legs as it moves up to your hips.

Now take a deep breath and slowly tighten the muscles in your abdomen and your lower back... hold them... and as you exhale... slowly release and relax completely...

Wonderful. With the next deep breath, tighten your middle and upper back muscles... hold them... and as you exhale, release and relax...

allow the area between your shoulder blades to relax even more...

Now... as you take a deep breath, tense the muscles in your shoulders and neck and hold... Very slowly release and relax... You may feel a light tingling sensation or feeling of warmth as the muscles release and relax. This is the area that we often need to relax even more, so take another deep breath... when you exhale, I want you to imagine that you are letting go of a heavy load that you have been carrying on your shoulders... as you let this load go, allow your shoulders to lower even more... you are releasing this load, you want to release... so go ahead, let it go... Good, very good.

As you inhale again, tighten the muscles in your chest and hold... and as you exhale, allow this beautiful feeling of relaxation to envelop your chest... relaxing your lungs, relaxing your heart, allowing your breathing to become more regular and more relaxed...

Bring your attention to your arms now and tighten the muscles in your upper arms, forearms, hands and fingers... make fists, if you wish, hold the tension for a while longer feeling it throughout your hands... and release... relax and release. Enjoy the wonderful feeling in your hands... so relaxed... so comfortable and so heavy...

Now let this wonderful feeling of relaxation flow right up into the back of your neck and into your head.

Please tighten the muscles in your head, hold... and relax... release and relax and as you relax... I want you to focus your attention on the muscles in your face.   Make a face. "Scrunch" up your face and tighten up the muscles... more... hold them... and relax. You may feel the movement of your facial muscles as they release and relax... The muscles of your forehead relax... the muscles of your eyes relax... the muscles around your eyes relax... the muscles of your cheeks relax... even your ears relax as the relaxation flows into your chin... Relax your teeth and all your body will relax much more... Let your jaw sag and all of your body muscles will go loose and limp, just as if you were a rag doll...

As you keep going deeper and deeper into this wonderful relaxed state... You have pleasant, contented thoughts going through your mind and wonderful, marvelous feelings flowing all throughout your entire body...

And now, we're going to tighten all the muscles together.
Begin now with your toes... feet... legs... stomach... back... hands... arms... chest... neck... shoulders... and face ... tighten ... hold ... and relax. Relax your body, relax your thoughts. Relax... relax. Good, very good.

You are going deeper and deeper into this wonderful relaxed state... where you have pleasant, contented thoughts going through your mind and wonderful, marvelous feelings flowing all throughout your entire body... And you just keep on going deeper and deeper as all the sounds around you send you deeper... Any sound that you may hear will send you deeper into calmness...

So as I keep on talking, you keep on relaxing... your mind relaxes as your body relaxes... with each and every breath you exhale, your body relaxes deeper... the beat of your heart keeps you going deeper... With each thought that you think, you are going deeper... Any sensation that you experience will drive you even deeper into this wonderful, comfortable, relaxed state... So allow your mind to guide you deeper... as I count from one down to five you will drift down deeper and your relaxation will double with each number you hear...

And you will find that the more you relax, the better you will feel, the better you feel, the more your body will relax...
And as your body relaxes, your mind will relax...

One...down... down... down... Your mind relaxes as your body relaxes, and your body doubles the relaxation that it has at this very moment...
Two... down... down... down... Your mind relaxes as your body relaxes, and your body doubles its

relaxation again... Three... down...down...down... your mind relaxes... Four... down... down... down... As your body relaxes... Five... down... down... down...

Another step down deeper, as your body again doubles its relaxation throughout your entire body... You feel warm, comfortable and relaxed as you keep going down deeper with each breath you exhale...

You feel wonderfully relaxed and comfortable as you float even deeper into this marvelous relaxed state, where your mind and body are now working together in perfect balance... Your mind is clear... Your muscles are loose and limp... Feel your nerves calm... Feel your blood flowing freely, carrying fresh new oxygen to all parts of your body... Feel your tissues rejuvenating in this wonderful relaxed state, as you go deeper and deeper...   And I would like you to go deeper, much deeper... so allow your mind to guide you even deeper...

Take a deep breath again - and as you exhale, let your entire body relax, as you go deeper and deeper into this wonderful relaxed state, just as if you were a rag doll... loose, limp and relaxed... deeper and deeper relaxed... Deeper, much deeper...

Drifting through this wonderful relaxed state... Going deeper with each breath you exhale... Now I am going to count from one down to ten... As I count from one down to ten, I want you to imagine, visualize, picture or just pretend that you are standing at the top of a stairway, with ten steps leading to a special, peaceful and beautiful place. You may even notice the blue sky above everything looking so soft and calm... Peaceful and pleasant.

You can imagine it to be any place you choose. Perhaps you would enjoy a beach or ocean with clean, fresh air... or the mountains with a stream... any place is perfectly fine...
In a moment you can begin to imagine taking a safe and gentle step down... down the stairway leading to a peaceful, special place for you, where you feel completely safe... comfortable... and secure.

With each step that you will take, you will find that, as your body relaxes, your mind relaxes... and with each step that you take, your body will triple its relaxation that it has at that time...

One... take the first step... Your mind relaxes as your body relaxes, and your body triples the relaxation that it has at this very moment... Two... take a second step... Your mind relaxes as your body relaxes, and your body triples its relaxation again... Three... another step. Your mind relaxes... Four... As your body relaxes... Five... Drifting down deeper, as your body again triples its relaxation... Six... Triples again... Seven... drifting down more and more... Eight... more and more relaxed... Nine... more and more

relaxed as you glide down... And ten... Deeper...
deeper... deeper... relaxed...
And now, imagine a peaceful and beautiful
place.

And as you mentally walk through this beautiful
place, touch the earth, what does it feel like?
Smell the air, what fragrances do you perceive?
What do you hear?
See it... smell it... touch it... Use all your senses!
Imagine yourself in this beautiful place......... and
feel that sense of peace flow through you... a
sense of safety and security.

Enjoy these positive feelings and keep them with
you long after this session is completed... for the
rest of this day, evening, and tomorrow...
Allow these positive feelings to grow stronger
and stronger... feeling at peace with a sense of
well being...
Each and every time that you are in this kind of
relaxation, you will be able to relax deeper and
deeper...

And these positive feelings will stay with you,
and grow stronger and stronger throughout the
day as you continue to relax deeper and deeper.
This is the most peaceful place in the world for
you... and as you move through this wonderful
place, find a comfortable place to sit and
perhaps even to lie down.

As you relax and let go, you notice that your mind opens up to welcome the helpful and beneficial suggestions.

You are deeply relaxed... you allow your mind to open up more and more.

Deeply relax. Each time in the future, when I say to you: *deeply relax...* your body will relax and you will sink deeply into this wonderful, comfortable, relaxed state. In this state, your body and mind are working together in perfect harmony, your mind is clear, your tissues are rejuvenating, and all you care about is how good you feel, how relaxed you feel, as you are enjoying the experience.

Deeply relax... you are instantly and spontaneously relaxing now into a wonderful calmness...
Your mind is clear and all you care about is enjoying the experience.

[Long pause.]

And now, slowly I will guide you back up to the point of full conscious awareness.

If you are in bed and want to fall asleep, all you need to do is take the headphones off or turn the player off and drift into a deep and restful sleep.... When it's time to wake up, you will awaken feeling wonderfully rejuvenated, full of energy and vitality, ready to enjoy another great day.

[Long pause.]

If you ready to be guided back up into full conscious awareness, I will count now from 5 up to number 1 - and will guide you into awakening.

When I reach number 1, you will open your eyes and feel wonderful, refreshed, energized and in very high spirits - feeling simply terrific.
5...
4...
3 - up, up, up, up ...
2 - feel the energies surging throughout your body awakening it completely!
1 - open your eyes!!! ... feeling great! ... Wonderfully Rejuvenated, full of energy and vitality... Ready to enjoy another great day!

==== END OF SCRIPT ====

I promise that if you do this for 21 days with consistency, you will be much closer to transforming your eating habits.

IS IT FUN YET?

STEP TWO - Weight Control

Now that you have listened to the Introduction to Deep Calmness, how do you feel?

Many people report suddenly feeling more in control, feeling "more together", and being able to see sharper colors. Many are able to sleep better at night and actually remember their dreams.

You may want to keep a dream diary, which can be as simple as a bedside notebook and pen, or the equivalent within arms' reach. Immediately upon awakening, write what you remember about your dream. This will jolt your dream recall and you may find that you start remembering more.

Sometimes, it's possible to gain reassurance or even answers to questions posed before sleep. (There's more about this in another book in my Calmness Series.)
Take time to notice how you feel. Notice the transformations that are happening. And remember the crucial importance of listening to this recording every day.

When you make a commitment to listen to this recording every day, you are making a commitment to better yourself and your life.

You are in control of your destiny by taking charge. What a wonderful feeling to be in control! How does it feel? In this state, you can accomplish anything you put your mind to.

==== **Start a journal** ====

Starting here I will be asking you to write your thoughts and feelings on several matters. I suggest you start a journal that you can refer back to later. This can even be a digital document, if that strikes your fancy.

=====================

Journey Within: Journal Entry

Please take just a few moments to consider the following questions and record your thoughts in your journal.

What would you like to achieve?
What goals and aspirations are coming to mind?

Take time to reflect and write them all down.

There are a few more topics to address before we introduce the second script. If we are going to revise your eating habits, let's first assess why you eat the way you do.

Ask Insightful Questions and Record Your Answers

Remember I said we need to take a journey inside?
Take a few deep breaths again.
Read through this section, then close your eyes and consider the following questions and thoughts.

Why do you eat the way you do?
What is your trigger?

Is it high fat foods? Is it sweets? Is it bread products? Why do you overeat? Are you under stress?

Some people find that they overeat when they are unhappy, tired, frustrated or simply bored. Still others overeat because they are numbing deep, internal pain.

Am I an Emotional Eater?

"I urgently need to eat - I crave a particular food and I feel a strong need to satisfy this craving even if it means going out late at night to get it." **When you are craving specific food, usually unhealthy food, it's a sign of emotional eating.**

"I am usually hungry after an argument." Physical hunger is not triggered by emotions. **If you find that you are hungry after an unsettling emotional situation that is most likely an emotional hunger.**

"I continue eating until my plate is empty." When you are eating because you are hungry, you will most likely stop eating when you are full. **Eating on auto-pilot (and not noticing how much you eat) is usually a sign of emotional eating.**

"I suddenly become hungry." Emotional hunger often comes on quickly and suddenly, physical hunger comes on gradually.

"I never feel satisfied, no matter how much I eat." Emotional hunger often demands more and more food to be satisfied. Physical hunger on the other hand doesn't need to be stuffed to feel satisfied.

"I feel disgusted or ashamed after eating." Feeling guilty after eating is a sign that part of you knows that you are not eating just to satisfy physical hunger.

"I think of food all the time and plan my day accordingly." Obsession with food can indicate emotional needs that are not met and that are transferred to constant thoughts of eating.

"I find that I eat unconsciously. Suddenly I am eating out of the ice cream container and soon after I discover that the whole container is empty." If you find that you are eating unconsciously, then most likely it's for emotional reasons, because if you eat for physical reasons you are usually aware of what you are doing.

During those brief moments when you are engrossed in eating, do you feel good, happy, or content?

Some people find that they're so busy at times they go all day without eating. Then, when they get home, they are often drawn to carbohydrates or sugar and feel that they "can't stop eating".
Others grew up feeling unloved, and this is their way of feeling or feeding the love.

Overcoming is the whole reason we're here! Discovering the triggers and effects is the first step to reworking any pattern.

Journey Within: Journal Entry

It is vital to understand the reasons you overeat. Take a few minutes now, put this book down, and write in your journal.

Write what you perceive are your reasons for overeating. Record the understandings you have gained as you've thought through what may be the triggering issues for your behaviors.

Consider your emotional state. Is it tranquil?
Consider your work circumstances. Are they peaceful?
Consider your schedule. Is it balanced? Are you eating the quick and easy food that's readily available: cookies, chocolate, cake, bread, pasta? Do you regularly forget to bring lunch to work, and end up running to McDonald's?

What is it that's causing the weight gain? You know it. You know the answer. Write it down. Put this book down, and write for five minutes.

Journey Within: Journal Entry

Now that you have been honest with yourself about your reasons for over-eating, you need to ask yourself why you wish to gain control of your weight.

Do you want to regain a more youthful appearance? Or do you want to create the healthiest body you possibly can?

Perhaps you just want to be healthy, respect yourself, and feed your body only wholesome, healthy foods? Or is there a particular reason for you to slim down – the approach of summer, a high school reunion or an upcoming wedding?

There is something very powerful about writing down your true desires, so I ask you to pull out your journal again.
Take a moment to write it down.

My reason for gaining control of my weight is...

Great! I'm so proud of you for progressing so far in the book. Please, give yourself a pat on the back for sticking with it!!
Although it's an easy process, you still needed to make the commitment, allocate the time and actually DO IT.

I know you've been wondering when we would finally get to the meat and potatoes of how to release excess weight and stay in control of your health! We've been laying a foundation and now you are ready to hear the weight mastery script. Again, this is a script that you need to record with a relaxed, calm, peaceful tone of voice, pausing whenever necessary.

As we've discussed previously, the retraining of your mind and creation of a new healthy habit will require at least 21 days. I trust that by now you are motivated to listen to this recording for at least 21 days. As you feel optimistic that this new recording can propel you forward toward a healthier, stronger, more youthful and more beautiful you, you are ready to optimize your success by listening to this recording daily for 21 days.

HEALTHY EATING

Do you consume high-fat, high-sugar snacks in between meals? *Or instead of meals*? Do you long for increased energy throughout the day? Do you desire to feel fit and productive? Then this first script is for you! In this highly effective script you are guided to restore feelings of health, energy and vitality. You are guided to release the desire for high-fat foods and sugars and to enjoy fruits and vegetables as healthy and life-giving snacks. As a result, you will find yourself more energized, feeling younger, healthier and stronger.

Ways to use this script:

As with the previous script, if you have a recording device available you may choose to record the following in your own voice. As a reminder: the script below should be recorded using a relaxed, peaceful and calming tone of voice, with pauses at the appropriate times. Keep space for some quiet time within the recording and be mindful to keep your words flowing smoothly. To help you relax even deeper, you may want to mix in peaceful relaxing music.

If you simply want to purchase a digital version that I've created and sold to people around the world, visit *calmness.com/wd* for an instant download.
For your convenience, I offer MP3s with voice only or with both voice and background music.

Weight Control – Healthy Eating script:

Take a deep breath and extend your arms up. Extend your stretch, pushing your arms out even further… feeling your spine stretch… Hold it for as long as it feels comfortable. And as you exhale, slowly lower your arms down… relaxing your body into complete limpness, like a rag doll… with your legs uncrossed… and your hands at your side or on your lap.

All you need now is to focus on a point of light. It can be any form of light, perhaps a glimmer on a piece of metal or even a bright object. Now… simply look toward the light, toward the source of brightness and allow your eyes to relax…
Allow the muscles around your eyes to relax and allow the muscles in your eyes to relax…
As you look toward the light… toward the source of brightness… Relax your eyes…

Simply allow the muscles <u>around</u> your eyes to relax and allow the muscles <u>in</u> your eyes to relax...

Continue looking toward the light, toward the source of brightness, until your eyes begin to grow heavy... then allow them to close... Simply allow your eyes to close........ Close your eyes and imagine the light... Imagine the source of brightness... Visualize it in your mind and allow your thoughts to relax...

Allow your body to relax... Relax, relax... and go deeper... Good... Now, I want you to take a deep breath... and let it out completely... relaxing your mind, relaxing your body... and sinking down into this comfortable, relaxed state.

I will be counting from 1 down to number 5 and with each and every number that I say, I would like you to take a deep breath, and each time I say the word "Relax", simply relax and allow the breath to flow out from your body...

One, take a deep breath... and relax... Two, take a deep breath... and relax... Three, take a deep, deep breath... and relax... Four, take a deep breath... and relax, release and relax... Five, take a deep, deep breath... and relax...

Relax your body, relax your thoughts as you allow this wonderful, comfortable feeling of relaxation flow all the way down to your feet... Good. Very good.

As you keep going deeper and deeper into this wonderful relaxed state... You have pleasant, contented thoughts going through your mind and wonderful, marvelous feelings flowing all throughout your entire body...

Relax your body, relax your thoughts. Relax... relax. Good, very good.

You are going deeper and deeper into this wonderful relaxed state... where you have pleasant, contented thoughts floating through your mind and wonderful, marvelous feelings flowing all throughout your entire body... And you just keep on going deeper and deeper as all the sounds around you send you deeper... Any sound that you may hear will send you deeper... So as I keep on talking, you keep on relaxing... your mind relaxes as your body relaxes... with each and every breath you exhale, your body relaxes deeper... the beat of your heart keeps you going deeper... With each thought that you think, you are going deeper... Any sensation that you experience will drive you even deeper into this wonderful, comfortable, relaxed state... So allow your mind to guide you deeper... as I count from one down to five you will drift down deeper and your relaxation will double with each number you hear...

And you will find that the more you relax, the better you will feel, the better you feel, the more your body will relax...
And as your body relaxes, your mind will relax...

One... down... down... down... Your mind relaxes as your body relaxes, and your body doubles the relaxation that it has at this very moment... Two... down... down... down... Your mind relaxes as your body relaxes, and your body doubles its relaxation again... Three... down... down... down... your mind relaxes... Four... down... down... down... As your body relaxes... Five... down... down... down... Another step down deeper, as your body again doubles its relaxation throughout your entire body... You feel warm, comfortable and relaxed as you keep going down deeper with each breath you exhale...

You feel wonderfully relaxed and comfortable as you float even deeper into this marvelous relaxed state, where your mind and body are now working together in perfect balance... Your mind is passive and clear... Your muscles are loose and limp... Feel your nerves calm... Feel your blood flowing freely, carrying fresh new oxygen to all parts of your body... Feel your tissues rejuvenating in this wonderful relaxed state, as you go deeper and deeper... And I want you to go deeper, much deeper... So allow your mind to guide you even deeper...

You find now that you feel so good... so comfortable... so relaxed...
You feel so good that all you care about is how good you feel, how relaxed you feel, as you drift deeper... so deep that your entire body has taken on a wonderful, comfortable, relaxed feeling... Your arms and legs feel so heavy, so comfortable and so relaxed... Your arms and legs

feel so comfortable, and so relaxed... you find that you are truly enjoying the experience.

Take a deep breath again... and as you exhale, let your entire body relax... as you go deeper and deeper into this wonderful relaxed state, just as if you were a rag doll... loose, limp and relaxed... deeper and deeper relaxed...
Deeper, much deeper...

Drifting through this wonderful calm state...
Relaxing deeper with each breath you exhale...
Now I am going to count from one down to ten...
As I count from one down to ten, I want you to imagine, visualize, picture, or just pretend that you are standing at the top of a stairway, with ten steps leading to a special, peaceful and beautiful place.
You may even notice the blue sky above everything looking so soft and calm... peaceful and pleasant...

You can imagine it to be any place you choose.
Perhaps you would enjoy a beach or ocean with clean, fresh air... or the mountains with a stream... Any place is perfectly fine...
In a moment you can begin to imagine taking a safe and gentle step down... down the stairway leading to a peaceful, special place for you, where you feel completely safe... comfortable... and secure.

With each step that you take, you will find that as your body relaxes, your mind relaxes... and with each step that you take, your body will triple its relaxation that it has at that time...

One... take a first step... Your mind relaxes as your body relaxes, and your body triples the relaxation that it has at this very moment... Two... take a second step... Your mind relaxes as your body relaxes, and your body triples its relaxation again... Three... your mind relaxes... Four... As your body relaxes... Five... Drifting down deeper, as your body again triples its relaxation... Six... Triples again... Seven... drifting down more and more... Eight... more and more relaxed... Nine... more and more relaxed as you glide down... And ten... Deeper... deeper... deeper... relaxed.

And now, imagine a peaceful and beautiful place...

And as you mentally walk through this beautiful place, touch the earth, what does it feel like? Smell the air, what fragrances do you perceive? What do you hear?

See it... smell it... touch it... Use all of your senses!

Imagine yourself in this beautiful place......... and feel that sense of peace flow through you... a sense of safety and security...

Enjoy these positive feelings and keep them with you long after this session is completed... for the rest of this day, evening, and tomorrow...

Allow these positive feelings to grow stronger and stronger... feeling at peace with a sense of well being.

Each and every time that you are in this kind of relaxation, you will be able to relax deeper and deeper...

And these positive feelings will stay with you, and grow stronger and stronger throughout the day as you continue to relax deeper and deeper.

This is the most peaceful place in the world for you... and as you move through this wonderful place, find a comfortable place to sit and perhaps even to lie down.

From this point forward, starting right now - you release all urges for high fat snacks between meals. Replace all those high fat, high sugar snacks with something good for you. Visualize yourself enjoying healthy snacks like fruits and vegetables. And as your in-between-meals snack, you see yourself eating apples, pears, bananas, oranges, melons, celery, carrots and other healthy and life-giving foods.
All desire to eat fattening, heavy, rich foods is draining away.

The inclination to have or eat such foods is leaving you now and is becoming like a distant memory... It is simply a past experience; it has no effect on you now.
You now release the desire to get high fat or sugar snacks between meals, because you are already full, you are completely satisfied by normal well-balanced meals.

Well-balanced meals... well-balanced, <u>moderate</u> meals <u>more</u> than satisfy your hunger. And the tastes of food are so sharp and clear that your appetite is satisfied, much more than before. The tastes of food fill you up and satisfy your hunger. You find that you enjoy food now more than you ever have before.

You savor the time that you take to eat; you savor the time that you take to eat. You <u>slow down</u> and enjoy the tastes, textures and fragrances of your food. You enjoy the tastes and fragrances of your food more than you ever have before. You feel good throughout the day, because your well-balanced meals have already satisfied your physical hunger... and also satisfied your mental appetite.
You stop eating once your hunger has been satisfied. You simply have no desire, urge or inclination to overeat.

You prefer to stop eating as soon as your hunger is gone... because you feel so much better, so much healthier, so much happier and more vigorous with a partially filled stomach. You completely <u>release</u> all desire to consume rich, heavy, greasy, sweet, fattening foods and drinks. You find that you are attracted to clean, healthy, life-giving foods and these healthy and nutritious foods taste and smell better than ever before!

Eating well-balanced meals helps you gain more energy. In fact, each day you awaken refreshed after a good night's rest. And with your newer and lighter figure, you will find that your energies have increased... and you feel stronger and healthier as you approach, and finally attain, your ideal weight and body.

Every time you exhale, the fat cells are evaporating and leaving your body... never to return again. And when you inhale, your body increases your elasticity and reshapes to its ideal size and form. Fat cells are melting away...

See the fat cells melting from specific areas on your body. See yourself breathing deeply throughout the day and knowing that it contributes to your increased metabolism.

Your body is releasing all the excess fat... The fat is released in a healthy, gentle way. You let go of the extra weight effortlessly, easily... You release the extra weight in a healthy way. You are becoming healthier and stronger as you achieve your ideal weight... And once you achieve your ideal weight, once you create the body you desire, you maintain that weight and body easily and effortlessly...

You are always aware of your eating. You now totally let go of any desire to eat when you are nervous, tense, frustrated, depressed, angry or bored. You have totally let go of any desire to eat when you are nervous, tense, frustrated, depressed, angry or bored.

[Long pause.]

I will count now from 5 up to number 1 - and will guide you into awakening.

When I reach number 1, you will open your eyes and feel wonderful, refreshed, energized and in very high spirits - feeling simply terrific.
5...
4...
3 - up, up, up, up ...
2 - feel the energies surging throughout your body awakening it completely!
1 - open your eyes!!! ... feeling great! ...
Wonderfully Rejuvenated, full of energy and vitality... Ready to enjoy another great day!

==== END OF SCRIPT ====

NIGHT EATER?

Do you feel the need to snack at night? Do you eat when watching television or reading a book? Do you feel hungry just a few short hours after dinner? I know that you are aware of how unhealthy snacking at night is for your body. In the next script you are encouraged to stop consumption of late night snacks and to embrace health. You are guided to become completely satisfied by a well-balanced moderate dinner while still increasing your energy levels!

Ways to use this script:

As with the previous script, if you have a recording device available you may choose to record the following in your own voice. The script below should be recorded using a relaxed, peaceful and calming tone of voice, with pauses at the appropriate times. Leave space for some quiet time within the recording and be mindful to keep your words flowing smoothly. To help you relax even deeper, you may want to mix in peaceful relaxing music.

If you want to simply purchase a digital version that I've created and sold to people around the world, visit *calmness.com/wn* for an instant download.

Weight Control - Control Night Snacking script:

Take a deep breath and extend your arms up. Extend your stretch, pushing your arms out even further... feeling your spine stretch... Hold it for as long as it feels comfortable. And as you exhale, slowly lower your arms down... relaxing your body into complete limpness, like a rag doll... with your legs uncrossed... and your hands on your side or on your lap.
All you need now is to focus on a point of light. It can be any form of light, perhaps a glimmer on a piece of metal or even a bright object.
Now... simply look toward the light, toward the source of brightness and allow your eyes to relax...

Allow the muscles around your eyes to relax and allow the muscles in your eyes to relax...
As you look toward the light... toward the source of brightness... relax your eyes...
Simply allow the muscles <u>around</u> your eyes to relax and allow the muscles <u>in</u> your eyes to relax...
Continue looking toward the light, toward the source of brightness, until your eyes begin to

grow heavy... then allow them to close... Simply allow your eyes to close....... Close your eyes and imagine the light... Imagine the source of brightness... Visualize it in your mind and allow your thoughts to relax...

Allow your body to relax... Relax, relax... and go deeper... Good... Now, I want you to take a deep breath... and let it out completely... relaxing your mind, relaxing your body... and sinking down into this comfortable, relaxed state.

I will be counting from 1 down to number 5 and with each and every number that I say, I would like you to take a deep breath, and each time I say the word "Relax", simply relax and allow the breath to flow out from your body...

One, take a deep breath... and relax... Two, take a deep breath... and relax... Three, take a deep, deep breath... and relax... Four, take a deep breath...and relax. Release and relax... Five, take a deep, deep breath... and relax...

Relax your body, relax your thoughts as you allow this wonderful, comfortable feeling of relaxation flow all the way down to your feet.... Good. Very good.

As you keep going deeper and deeper into this wonderful relaxed state... You have pleasant, contented thoughts going through your mind and wonderful, marvelous feelings flowing all throughout your entire body...

Relax your body, relax your thoughts. Relax… relax. Good, very good.

You are going deeper and deeper into this wonderful relaxed state… where you have pleasant, contented thoughts floating through your mind and wonderful, marvelous feelings flowing all throughout your entire body… And you just keep on going deeper and deeper… as all the sounds around you send you deeper… Any sound that you may hear will send you deeper…

So as I keep on talking, you keep on relaxing… your mind relaxes as your body relaxes… with each and every breath you exhale, your body relaxes deeper… the beat of your heart keeps you going deeper… With each thought that you think, you are going deeper… Any sensation that you experience will guide you even deeper into this wonderful, comfortable, relaxed state… So allow your mind to guide you deeper… as I count from one down to five you will drift down deeper and your relaxation will double with each number you hear…

And you will find that the more you relax, the better you will feel… the better you feel, the more your body will relax…
And as your body relaxes, your mind will relax…

One… down… down… down… Your mind relaxes as your body relaxes, and your body doubles the relaxation that it has at this very moment…

Two… down… down… down… Your mind relaxes as your body relaxes, and your body doubles its relaxation again… Three… down… down… down… your mind relaxes… Four… down… down… down… As your body relaxes… Five… down… down… down… Another step down deeper, as your body again doubles its relaxation throughout your entire body… You feel warm, comfortable and relaxed as you keep going down deeper with each breath you exhale…

You feel wonderfully relaxed and comfortable as you float even deeper into this marvelous relaxed state… where your mind and body are now working together in perfect balance… Your mind is passive and clear… Your muscles are loose and limp… Feel your nerves calm… Feel your blood flowing freely, carrying fresh new oxygen to all parts of your body… Feel your tissues rejuvenating in this wonderful relaxed state, as you go deeper and deeper… And I want you to go deeper, much deeper… so allow your mind to guide you even deeper…

You find now that you feel so good… so comfortable… so relaxed…
You feel so good that all you care about is how good you feel, how relaxed you feel, as you drift deeper… so deep that your entire body has taken on a wonderful, comfortable, relaxed feeling… Your arms and legs feel so heavy, so comfortable and so relaxed… Your arms and legs feel so comfortable, and so relaxed… that you find you are truly enjoying the experience.

Take a deep breath again - and as you exhale, let your entire body relax... as you go deeper and deeper into this wonderful relaxed state, just as if you were a rag doll... loose, limp and relaxed... deeper and deeper relaxed... Deeper, much deeper...

Drifting through this wonderful calm state... Relaxing deeper with each breath you exhale... Now I am going to count from one down to ten... As I count from one down to ten, I want you to imagine, visualize, picture or just pretend that you are standing at the top of a stairway, with ten steps leading to a special, peaceful and beautiful place. You may even notice the blue sky above everything looking so soft and calm... Peaceful and pleasant...

You can imagine it to be any place you choose. Perhaps you would enjoy a beach or ocean with clean, fresh air... or the mountains with a stream... any place is perfectly fine...
In a moment you can begin to imagine taking a safe and gentle step down... down the stairway leading to a peaceful, special place for you, where you feel completely safe... comfortable... and secure.

With each step that you will take, you will find that, as your body relaxes, your mind relaxes... and with each step that you take, your body will triple its relaxation that it has at that time...

One... take a first step... Your mind relaxes as your body relaxes, and your body triples the relaxation that it has at this very moment... Two... take a second step... Your mind relaxes as your body relaxes, and your body triples its relaxation again... Three... your mind relaxes... Four... As your body relaxes... Five... Drifting down deeper, as your body again triples its relaxation... Six... Triples again... Seven... drifting down more and more... Eight... more and more relaxed... Nine... more and more relaxed as you glide down... And ten... Deeper... deeper... deeper... relaxed...

And now, imagine a peaceful and beautiful place...

And as you mentally walk through this beautiful place, touch the earth, what does it feel like? Smell the air, what fragrances do you perceive? What do you hear?

See it... smell it... touch it... Use all your senses! Imagine yourself in this beautiful place......... and feel that sense of peace flow through you... a sense of safety and security...

Enjoy these positive feelings and keep them with you long after this session is completed... for the rest of this day, evening, and tomorrow...

Allow these positive feelings to grow stronger and stronger... feeling at peace with a sense of well being...

Each and every time that you are in this kind of relaxation, you will be able to relax deeper and deeper...

And these positive feelings will stay with you, and grow stronger and stronger throughout the day as you continue to relax deeper and deeper. This is the most peaceful place in the world for you... and as you move through this wonderful place, find a comfortable place to sit and perhaps even to lie down.

From this point forward, starting right now - you release all urges for late night snacks. All desire to eat fattening, heavy, rich foods is draining away. The inclination to have or eat such foods is leaving you now and is becoming like a distant memory... It is simply a past experience; it has no effect on you now.

You now release the desire to get a late night snack, because you are already full, you are completely satisfied by normal well-balanced dinner. You eat well-balanced meals... well-balanced, moderate meals and they more than satisfy your hunger. The tastes of food are so sharp and clear that your appetite is satisfied, more than ever before. The tastes of food fill you up and satisfy your hunger. You find that you enjoy food now more than ever before.

You will savor the time that you take to eat; you savor the time that you take to eat. You slow down and enjoy the tastes, textures and fragrances of your food. You enjoy the tastes and fragrances of your food more than you ever have before. You feel good throughout the day... because your well-balanced meals have already satisfied your physical hunger and your mental appetite. You stop eating once your hunger has been satisfied.

You prefer to stop eating as soon as your hunger is gone - because you feel so much better, so much healthier, so much happier and more vigorous with a partially-filled stomach. You completely release all desire to consume rich, heavy, greasy, sweet, fattening foods and drinks. You find that you are attracted to clean, healthy, life-giving foods... these healthy and nutritious foods taste better and smell better than ever before.

Eating well-balanced meals helps you gain more energy. In fact, each day you awaken refreshed after a good night's rest. And with your newer and lighter body, you find that your energies have increased... You feel stronger and healthier as you approach and <u>finally attain</u> your ideal weight and body.

Every time you exhale, the fat cells are evaporating and leaving your body - never to return again. And when you inhale, your body increases your elasticity and reshapes to its ideal size and form. Fat cells are melting away...

See the fat cells melting and evaporating from your body... See yourself breathing deeply throughout the day and knowing that it contributes to your increased metabolism.

Your body is releasing all the excess fat. The fat is released in a healthy, gentle way. You release the extra weight in a healthy way... You are becoming healthier and stronger as you achieve your ideal weight. And once you achieve your ideal weight, once you create the body you desire, you maintain that weight and body... effortlessly, easily.

You are <u>always</u> aware of your eating. You now totally let go of any desire to eat when you are nervous, tense, frustrated, depressed, angry or bored. You have totally let go of any desire to eat when you are nervous, tense, frustrated, depressed, angry or bored.

[Long pause.]

If you ready to be guided back up into full conscious awareness, I will count now from 5 up to number 1 - and will guide you into awakening.

When I reach number 1, you will open your eyes and feel wonderful, refreshed, energized and in very high spirits - feeling simply terrific.
5...
4...
3 - up, up, up, up ...
2 - feel the energies surging throughout your body awakening it completely!

1 - open your eyes!!! … feeling great! … Wonderfully Rejuvenated, full of energy and vitality… Ready to enjoy another great day!

==== END OF SCRIPT ====

Suddenly, the quest for a true happy state of mind becomes completely reachable, as calmness reprograms your inner computer.

You realize that you are capable of taking charge and that you possess great tools for self-improvement!

Weight Control Script Response

Journey Within: Journal Entry

Now that you've listened to all the powerful and positive guided imagery scripts, how wonderful do you feel? How empowered do you feel? Take this time to write down how you feel and be inspired to use big, potent words like: fabulous, powerful, remarkable, ecstatic, energetic, accomplished, optimistic, enthusiastic, peaceful...

I am committed to taking charge of my mind, body, and spirit.

I am excited that you have progressed so far and are ready for the next step! You are ready to eat healthy, to take care of your body, and to take better control of your life. The benefits are enormous!

* Increased self-esteem,
* Ability to stay calm and in balance,
* Stronger, more youthful body and mind,
* Powerful immune system and quicker healing,
* Positive outlooks on life and vitality,
   and most of all ...
            ... a Happier You!

MAINTAINING THE RIGHT THOUGHTS

STEP THREE – Your Daily Practice

Mahatma Gandhi said, "A man is but the product of his thoughts. What he thinks, he becomes." Throughout the day your mind is constantly at work, dictating choices that you make. In this final script, you will find positive constructive affirmations that you can say throughout the day to express your commitment to achieving and maintaining a healthy, lean, strong, thin body. Record this script separately, and listen to it throughout the day. Be sure to record the affirmations (on the next page) with pauses after each phrase, so that when you are listening to them you can repeat each phrase *after you hear it spoken on the recording*.

Or to simply purchase the digital version of these affirmations and receive an instant download visit calmness.com/wd
Choose the Affirmations option on the drop-down menu. To help optimize your results, the digital versions include 3 audible and 3 subliminal recordings.

Affirmations - Weight Control

I am enjoying well-balanced moderate meals.
I like healthy snacks.
I drink plenty of water.
I enjoy the tastes of fruits and vegetables.
I feel good throughout the day.
I eat small meals.
I am satisfied with less food.
I eat a wide variety of fruits and vegetables throughout the day.
I eat slowly.
I take small bites.
I chew my food thoroughly.
I savor every bite of food.
I stop eating when my hunger is satisfied.
I stop eating long before I am full.
I enjoy large glasses of fresh water.
People are much more attracted to me already.
As the days progress, I feel stronger and healthier.
I release all excess fat.
I release all desire to consume fats and sweets.
I visualize the ideal figure for my height and bone structure.
My body is being shaped according to my liking
I enjoy my body.
I am becoming healthier and stronger as I achieve my ideal figure.
The fat is melting away as it is consumed by my body.
I enjoy exercising to help my body consume the fat.

My hips and thighs are becoming smaller, as the fat is consumed.
My stomach is becoming flatter, as the fat is consumed.
I release all urges for late night snacks.
I feel completely satisfied with my dinner.
I am free from any need or desire to eat late in the evening.
All the fat is disappearing from the right areas.
I wake up in the morning feeling alive!

==== END OF SCRIPT ====

Are you wondering what became of my shy friend, who called wanting to release 300 pounds?

Through further conversations, I found out the person on the phone was a male. Obesity had reduced his testosterone level to the point of his voice sounding genderless. At first Robert and I needed to work together over the phone, as he was afraid to leave his home. His agoraphobia gripped him with anxiety, he had difficulty sleeping through the night while dealing with sleep apnea, and he also found himself continuously eating, never feeling satisfied.

We had a few phone sessions in which I helped him overcome his phobia, and then we began to meet in person to take charge of his health and weight. After we started working together, his determination to *finally heal* grew and despite many challenges, he completed the program. I followed up with Robert two years after and he is much happier and doing well! He remarried and is running a successful online business. He is at a healthy weight (under 200 pounds) and maintaining it with ease. I am so proud of how far he has gone in pursuit of life satisfaction. **The techniques and scripts we used are the same as those available in this book for you!**

Dear Friend, I'm happy that you've come this far! I am glad that you are committed to your success and that you are ready to get on the road to a better you.

Other people are greatly encouraged by stories of success. Please share your journey, as you never know whom it might help.
I would love to hear your success story! Please share it with us at calmness.com/weight

Visit calmness.com!
Subscribe to the e-newsletter for Free Gifts and to receive more encouragement, techniques, and guidance to support you on your journey.

What else?

So what else would you like to accomplish?
Would you like to be financially independent?
Would you like to be able to sleep better?
How about meeting the love of your life or improving your relationships?
Or maybe quitting smoking?
Do you want to let go of your anger or guilt?
Would you like to improve your memory?
Do you want to stop biting your nails?
Would you like to increase your self-esteem?
Would you like to develop your spirituality?

Check out other books in this series, and choose the subject that you want to tackle next.
Enjoy your life!!!

Check in often, as we're regularly adding other titles.

Yours in calmness,

Dr. Inessa

PERSONAL GUIDANCE

Recordings are available to facilitate personal development in the privacy of you home.

Visit: calmness.com

Dr. Inessa conducts group training seminars and individual coaching in person, over the phone, and through Skype.
.
For Hosting or Speaking Appearances please visit:
http://calmness.com/go/contact

For Coaching and/or Consulting, please contact:
Dr.Inessa@calmness.com

REFERENCES

[1] http://www.who.int/mediacentre/factsheets/fs311/en/

[2] http://www.win.niddk.nih.gov/statistics/

[3] http://www.hsph.harvard.edu/obesity-prevention-source/obesity-consequences/economic/

[4] http://www.hsph.harvard.edu/obesity-prevention-source

[5] McGinnis JM, Foege WH (1993) Actual causes of death in the United States. JAMA 270: 2207–2212.

[6] http://preventcancer.aicr.org/site/News2?page=NewsArticle&id=9639&news_iv_ctrl=0&abbr=res_&gclid=CMeJuYzzqLsCFUjxOgodM2gAkQ

[7] http://stanfordhospital.org/clinicsmedServices/COE/surgicalServices/generalSurgery/bariatricsurgery/obesity/effects.html

[8] http://www.hopkinsmedicine.org/digestive_weight_loss_center/conditions/diabetes.html

[9] http://circ.ahajournals.org/content/96/9/3248.full

[10] http://www.nhlbi.nih.gov/health/public/heart/chol/wyntk.htm

[11] http://www.nejm.org/doi/full/10.1056/NEJMoa021423

[12] Clark AM, Ledger W, Galletly C, et al. Weight loss results in significant improvement in pregnancy and ovulation rates in anovulatory obese women. *Hum Reprod*. 1995;10(10):2705-2712.

[13] http://bjp.sagepub.com/content/early/2013/04/08/2049463713484296.full

[14] http://www.medscape.com/viewarticle/564201_6

[15] http://www.ncbi.nlm.nih.gov/pmc/articles/PMC3063914/

[16] http://www.ncbi.nlm.nih.gov/pubmed/11192327

[17] http://www.ncbi.nlm.nih.gov/pubmed/22078437

[18] http://www.ncbi.nlm.nih.gov/pubmed/12080440

[19] http://www.ncbi.nlm.nih.gov/pubmed/18796104

[20] http://www.mayoclinic.org/news2012-mchi/6759.html

[21] http://www.ncbi.nlm.nih.gov/pubmed/23025954

[22] http://www.mayoclinic.com/health/erectile-dysfunction/DS00162/DSECTION=risk-factors

[23] http://www.ncbi.nlm.nih.gov/pmc/articles/PMC2866035/

[24] http://jasn.asnjournals.org/content/17/6/1695.full

[25] http://www.cancer.gov/cancertopics/pdq/supportivecare/lymphedema/healthprofessional

[26] http://www.mayoclinic.com/health/cellulitis/DS00450/DSECTION=risk-factors

[27] http://www.nlm.nih.gov/medlineplus/ency/article/000085.htm

[28] http://www.medscape.com/viewarticle/718012

[29] http://www.mayoclinic.com/health/osteoarthritis/DS00019/DSECTION=risk-factors

[30] http://www.medscape.com/viewarticle/747967

www.ingramcontent.com/pod-product-compliance
Lightning Source LLC
Chambersburg PA
CBHW070306290526
45791CB00003B/1097